THE OSTEOPENIA HANDBOOK

Beat It with Healthy Bones

*Differences Between Osteopenia & Osteoporosis,
Ways to Prevent and Treat, 20+ Risk Factors for
Both Men & Women, Commonly Prescribed
Medications, and More!*

ELIZABETH GRAY

Printed in the United States of America

First Printing, 2018

ISBN-13:
978-1721035441

ISBN-10:
1721035443

Elizabeth Gray Publishing
18 Key Street
Millis, MA 02054

In Hollywood, you play a mom and instantly, you've got osteoporosis.

- GABRIELLE UNION

DISCLAIMER

The information in this book does not contain medical professional advice. Individuals requiring such services should consult a competent medical professional. The author makes no representations about the suitability of the information contained in this book for any purpose. This material is provided "as is" and this publication is for informational purposes only.

Table
OF CONTENTS

Introduction

I'm writing this because a friend, who is very healthy, has been diagnosed with osteopenia. I never knew this was the step before osteoporosis and as my other friend says, "We all have it." Being fairly young, I wanted this condition to not turn in osteoporosis! I had no desire to be one of those hunched over ladies or as is becoming more common these days, to have a hip replacement.

Can osteopenia be cured or not move on to become the dreaded osteoporosis? I decided to do my own research to find out as much as I could because I remember my mom saying when she was in her eighties that she stopped taking a common drug for osteoporosis called Fosamax because it made her sick to her stomach. She never became hunched over and fortunately never had any sort of hip replacement surgery. She may be just lucky or maybe she subconsciously knew something. And did she ever get diagnosed with osteopenia? I don't know because she kept her medical issues private and now both my parents have passed.

Once again, I decided to research the subject to the best of my ability for I am not a nurse or a doctor. But I have worked in the medical field and know the best patient is educated on various treatment options and preventative care. Patients need to know this information not only for themselves but they need to know the right questions to ask of their doctor. Especially when other medications you may be taking may be good for your general health but bad for your bone health.

So, my hope is that this book will put the information on osteopenia together and it will help you whatever your osteopenia degree is. Or it will help you learn too if you are just curious on how you can prevent an osteopenia diagnosis for yourself or a loved one.

What Is Osteopenia Anyway and Its Difference from Osteoporosis?

First of all osteopenia it is not a disease. Sometimes people think of osteopenia as being somewhere between having healthy bones and osteoporosis. Osteopenia means bone mineral density (BMD) is below normal levels but not low enough to be qualified as osteoporosis. Osteopenia and osteoporosis are related. Both are varying degrees of bone loss, as measured by bone mineral density (BMD), a marker for how strong a bone is and the risk that it might break. Osteopenia, which affects about half of Americans over age 50, is sometimes the precursor to osteoporosis.

Osteoporosis is considered to be a bone disease. According to the National Osteoporosis Foundation, the definition of osteoporosis is "a bone disease that occurs when the body loses too much bone, makes too little bone, or both." Their research says about 54 million people in the United States have osteoporosis. In fact, if you live long enough, you might get osteoporosis. Aging means our bone material is naturally not replaced as quickly as when we were young. Many people have been diagnosed with osteopenia but they never come down with osteoporosis. Why?

With the osteopenia disorder, your bones are not at the breaking point but they are weaker than normal. It occurs when bones become weaker and are less "dense." It is a warning sign that your bones are becoming more fragile and are more prone to breaks.

Bones are at their densest usually at age 30. This density keeps lessening after that age and bones get less dense as you age. Strong bones depend on your diet to get the nutrients they need to grow and be healthy. Minerals that your bones need include: calcium, phosphorus, magnesium, potassium, and zinc. If there are not enough minerals that bones need, the rate of bone formation decreases and bone loss increases. Thereby causing weak bones. Osteopenia raises your risk of a bone fracture because the more porous your bones are the more likely they are to break. But because people with osteopenia have higher bone mineral density (BMD) than those with osteoporosis, the risk of a fracture is lower for people with osteopenia.

A sedentary life style or inactive life can weaken your bones. Certain habits like too much alcohol, caffeine or not drinking enough water can also weaken your bones.

However, I want to stress, having osteopenia does not mean it will automatically turn into osteoporosis. Diet, exercise and sometimes medication can make a difference. Start now and talk to your doctor about the proper diet and exercise plan to stop it from becoming osteoporosis.

But before we jump ahead I need to explain what a bone exactly is. A medical definition is: "Bone is the substance that forms the skeleton of the body. It is composed chiefly of calcium phosphate and calcium carbonate. It also serves as a storage area for calcium, playing a large role in calcium balance in the blood."

Bone is living tissue. A bone's cells, nerves, blood and minerals are always renewing themselves. In fact, cells in the skeletal system regenerate almost constantly, but the complete process takes a full 10 years. This renewal process slows down as we age, so our bones get thinner. Your body is constantly losing old bone and forming new bone, but as you get older, your body is unable to make new bone at the same rate that old bone is lost. This sometimes means osteopenia unless you take action to prevent it.

Low bone density means that you don't have healthy bone density to keep our bones strong or "dense." With low bone density we may have difficulty in supporting our body weight and protect our internal organs to help us to move. The weaker the bones as well, the easier they are to break.

Osteopenia is a bone condition characterized by a decreased density of bone, which leads to bone weakening and an increased risk of breaking a bone (fracture).
Other types too of weak bone conditions exist. Osteomalacia, osteomyelitis, and osteoarthritis are different conditions that cause bones to be weak and more prone to fracture.

Osteopenia does not cause any pain unless a bone is broken or fractured. But even so, fractures do not always cause pain so osteopenia (or even osteoporosis) can be present for many years prior to any diagnosis.

In your younger years, you probably took your bones for granted. That is until something happens to them! To protect yourself from a fracture or a bone disease like osteoporosis, it's essential to eat a nutrient dense diet and have other healthy lifestyle habits such as doing weight-bearing exercises. If your bones are dense and strong you may never get osteopenia. Or osteoporosis. So if you haven't been diagnosed yet, now might the time to incorporate healthy habits to prevent ever getting osteopenia.

Who Is Most Likely to Get Osteopenia and What Is Its Symptoms?

There are usually no symptoms. Much like high blood pressure that is the "silent killer." You notice no pain or change when your bones become thinner. If you fracture a bone your doctor may diagnose you with osteopenia. For example, if you are above 50, and you break a bone after a fall, you may be likely to have weak bones and osteopenia. You are losing more bone than you are creating.

A sign might occur if you're suffering from one or more bone fractures or breaks; you have pain and aches affecting tissues near the bone (this includes joint pain); and you have trouble exercising due to pain.

You should tell your doctor too if you have a family history of osteoporosis. And if you are thin, Caucasian, Asian, don't exercise, are a smoker, drink alcohol in excess, and even if you consume soda regularly might mean you are at a higher risk to get osteopenia. If you have an eating disorder or metabolism problem the body may not get enough vitamins or minerals to build strong bones. If you've used corticosteroids, such as prednisone or hydrocortisone, on a long term basis for inflammatory conditions or anticonvulsants for pain or seizures you could be in jeopardy of having osteopenia.

Also, chemotherapy can increase your risk. If you've been inactive or bedridden for a long time or you have a diet low in calcium or vitamin D (you must have vitamin D in order to absorb calcium and prevent bone loss) you may have osteopenia. Talk to your doctor if any of these hold true.

How Is Osteopenia Diagnosed?

Without any symptoms, how is osteopenia diagnosed by a doctor?

If you have risk factors, your physician will recommend a bone mineral density test, the most accurate being a dual-energy X-ray absorptiometry or DXA scan. DXA is a form of X-ray to detect bone loss. It involves using a low-energy X-ray that assesses the level of calcium in bones. A regular X-ray is not adequate because it is not sensitive enough.

The National Osteoporosis Foundation suggests that the best places to perform the test are the hip or spine. This is where people usually get fractures.

The test results use a T-score. A t score compares bone mineral density to a reference mean. To give you an example, a normal T-score is above -1.0. Osteopenia is diagnosed with a T-score between -0.1 to -2.5. The test itself is painless and fast.

T-score	Diagnosis
+1.0 to –1.0	normal bone density
–1 to –2.5	low bone density, or osteopenia
–2.5 or more	osteoporosis

Standard screening for osteoporosis is recommended for women over age 65. And women ages 60 to 64 should be screened if they've gone through menopause and have at least one risk factor. As both women and men age, your bones naturally become weaker. Women over age 50 and men over age 70 have a higher risk of osteoporosis. In women, the drop in estrogen at menopause is a major cause of bone loss; in men, a drop in testosterone can cause bone loss. Unfortunately, women do have a greater chance than men of developing osteopenia and later, osteoporosis, because of their lower peak BMD. The loss of bone mass spreads out too as hormonal changes take place during menopause.

If a T-score shows you have osteopenia, your DXA report may include your FRAX (Fracture Risk Assessment Tool) score. If it doesn't, your doctor can calculate it for you. The FRAX tool uses your bone density and other risk factors to estimate your risk of breaking your hip, spine, forearm, or shoulder within the next ten years. Your doctor may also use your FRAX score to help make decisions about treatment for osteopenia. Once again, your bones are frail but not as frail as they would be with osteoporosis.

But if you're younger than 60, speak to a medical professional about your specific medical condition and concerns. For example, teens and college-age women who are thin and who exercise excessively are at a high risk of not having menstrual periods. This is called amenorrhea. Loss of menstrual periods is linked to decreased estrogen levels. Decreased levels of estrogen may cause bone loss. A diet low in calcium and other bone-boosting nutrients can also contribute to low bone density. Teenage girls who restrict their eating and who lack menstrual periods are even at risk of osteoporosis and fractures! Way past having osteopenia. Or young female athletes try to reach a low body weight. They appear to be in top physical condition but they are often at risk for a fracture. This can alert your doctor that someone may have osteopenia and suggest they have a bone density test.

If your doctor decides you should have the test, you may need a referral or insurance may not pay for it. Most health insurers will pay for the test if you've had a fracture; you've been through menopause; you're not taking estrogen at menopause; you take medications that cause bone thinning. You may want to check with your insurance company before you have the test done to see if they will cover it.

So, always discuss with your doctor if you should have the test. And remember, some people who have osteopenia may not have significant bone loss. They may just naturally have a lower bone density. Your doctor will evaluate your medical condition and if you should even worry!

As we move into the future, osteopenia can and should be prevented. For not too long ago, osteoporosis was thought to be a natural part of aging. Most medical professionals agree that this is no longer true. So, it follows, humans do not naturally get osteopenia. This health disorder can be totally prevented or absolutely lessened.

Risk Factors

Early detection of low bone mass is the most important step for prevention and treatment. If you don't know you have it, you can't treat it! Your doctor will take a medical history and may decide you need a bone density test if one or more of the following risk factors pertain. Tell the doctor immediately if a loss of height, change in posture (a stoop or hunched back), or sudden back pain is noticed. This can indicate a vertebral fracture…a fracture of the spine. And mean you already have osteoporosis. The more risk factors you have as well, the more chances you have to get osteopenia.

Risk factors for osteopenia include:

- Being a woman having gone through menopause. The hormonal changes such as lower estrogen can contribute to a low bone density. Estrogen is important in maintaining strong, healthy bones. Having strong bones is critical before menopause. You might want to tell any daughters…even teen-aged and younger…to follow healthy habits for strong bones now!

- Eating a diet low in calcium and vitamin D. Vitamin D helps in absorbing calcium. Some people need to avoid all dairy products whether by choice (vegetarians or vegans) or because of a medical condition (lactose intolerant). But calcium is found in vegetables too.

- We have all heard about Vitamin D deficiency. The best way to prevent this is to expose your bare skin to sunlight for about 15 to 20 minutes a day. This means going without sunscreen! You should definitely use it after that to do any outdoor activity. To avoid the risk of cancer. But staying indoors most of the time and avoiding the sun completely may mean your body isn't making the vitamin D it needs.

However, the 15 to 20 minutes a day is a rough estimate. Many factors can interfere with vitamin D synthesis. People with dark skin need two to three times the sun exposure to make the same amount of vitamin D as those with light skin. Synthesis declines with age as well. Clouds, ozone and air pollution can decrease vitamin D production too. Supplements can help but are not the same as going outdoors. The recommend dosage is 600 IU of vitamin D per day but speak to your doctor if you need more or less. Also, vitamin D can be found in food such as salmon and fortified foods.

- Having an eating disorder, such as anorexia or bulimia, or undereating for many years. This means a person's body is not getting the necessary nutrients for strong, healthy bones. This can occur in both men and women but happens to women more. Low body fat can decrease hormones such as estrogen. Eating disorders can develop in early adolescence when the skeleton is in the process of growing. This can mean osteopenia or even osteoporosis in women as young as in their early 20's.

- Having a sedentary lifestyle or not getting enough exercise. Most of us know by now that weight-bearing exercise is important and helps bones to maintain their strength.

- Taking some medications can weaken bones such as steroids to treat asthma. They can interfere with the body's mineral levels such as calcium. Also chemotherapy can interfere and too much exposure to radiation.

- Having certain medical condition such as lupus, rheumatoid arthritis, and celiac disease also increases your chances of having osteopenia. If you have an overactive thyroid, too much thyroid medication can also play a role. Graves' disease can result in an overactive thyroid. And if any thyroid condition is treated with a thyroxine hormone, there is some concern that an over replacement may impact bone health.

- Having an illness or disease with their treatments can affect bone strength such as chronic liver disease, chronic kidney disease, or Coeliac disease.

- Experiencing breast cancer. Women with breast cancer have an increased risk even of developing osteoporosis because of the treatments used and their effect on estrogen levels. Speak to your oncologist about having a bone density test done.

- Having rheumatoid arthritis. It's an inflammatory disease which primarily attacks flexible joints. It's a condition affecting many in the general population. Also, if prednisolone is prescribed, this can lead to the development of osteoporosis.

- Being a Caucasian or Asian may be a risk factor. Also a factor might be being thin or having a family history of osteoporosis. Especially if you've have a parent or sibling who has had a hip fracture.

- Being inactive or bedridden for a long time.

- Drinking excessive amounts of alcohol or caffeine. Alcohol inhibits the absorption of minerals by reducing your levels of magnesium. Coffee increases the rate of calcium and magnesium excretion by urine. If you drink more than two cups of coffee a day, you increase your risk of breaking bones.

- Avoid stress! Easier said than done in today's society. But it's important not only for your bone health but general health. Stress interferes with your adrenal gland with will lead to low production of serotonin and an increase in cortisol. High levels of cortisol will make you not sleep. When you're asleep new tissues and bones will form. So avoid stress and get enough sleep!

- And of course, smoking, is a big risk factor. Smoking causes a significant reduction in bone density and often women can experience menopause earlier (approximately two years).

Is Osteopenia Risk for Men?

A ll people over the age of 50 are at an increased risk of developing osteopenia. But women are at a much higher risk than men. Their bones are usually smaller and thinner than men's. And estrogen plays a role in bone reabsorption and new bone growth. In menopause, estrogen decreases and the risk for osteopenia increases.

Osteopenia, and if it develops, osteoporosis, are very common. Statistics show that people with osteopenia do tend to develop osteoporosis but it can be prevented. And even though the risks are higher for women, men can come down with osteopenia or osteoporosis as well. Many men believe that it's just "an old woman's disease." But since the research on men is limited, men are more likely to get osteopenia due to lifestyle factors like smoking, drinking, or taking a medication that increases the risk of bone loss, such as some antidepressants and corticosteroids.

Corticosteroids are man-made drugs that work like a natural hormone in your body to reduce inflammation and alter the immune system. They treat medical conditions such as arthritis, asthma, allergies, skin conditions, autoimmune diseases, inflammatory bowel diseases, and cancer.

And even though bone loss in men occurs much later in life compared to when it develops in women, by age 65 men catch up to women losing the same amount of bone. In fact, it's estimated that by 2025, the total number of hip fractures will be the same in men and women.

The following risk factors for men are true for many women as well.

- Your genes and ethnic background. Your natural body type could determine whether you have a small, medium, or large bone structure. Those with a smaller bone structure are men usually of Asian, Indian and Caucasian descent. People of African-American and Hispanic descent, have a tendency towards much higher bone density.

- Eating too many processed and sugary foods is more common in men. Not only is there a lack of nutritional value in them but that also leech calcium from your bones. From overly-salty snacks to high-in-sugar sodas, certain foods can inhibit your body from absorbing calcium and thus reduce bone mineral density.

- Exercising too much! Yes, exercise is good for you but too much of it is not a good thing. Just like when you are injured if you put excessive stress on muscles, the same can occur with your bones. We need some stress to maintain strength, but if you're exercising too much you could be putting your bones at risk.

- Not diversifying your workout routine. Running and jogging are good for bone density but this should be alternated with exercises like barbell deep back squats and military presses. These are great to work out some of the largest muscle/bone groups in the body.

- Too much smoking and drinking. Excessive alcohol intake can reduce the absorption of minerals and vitamins and can decrease bone growth and smoking also manipulates hormones responsible for mineralizing bone.

- Taking steroids. Use of steroids (including prescription steroidal medications) are related to bone density.

- Smoking marijuana? Research is still in its infancy on whether this drug hurts or helps bone loss. As research has shown, smoking tobacco is very detrimental to bone health because of the nicotine. Nicotine causes vascular constriction, limiting the blood flow to the bones. But there is no nicotine in marijuana. Studies show that heavy users generally have a lower body weight and body mass index (BMI) than non-users...factors associated with bone thinning. So is marijuana bad for bones? This may become more of a concern as states continue to legalize its use for medicinal or recreational purposes. If you are using marijuana, discuss bone density with your doctor and seen if you might need an assessment.

Medical research on men is still very limited and is often not recognized. But if a man falls in a parking lot and causes a hip to be broken, that may be their first symptom of osteopenia...or even osteoporosis. Because men have higher bone density than women at middle age osteopenia happens at an older age for men than women. Men also don't go through menopause. But men are at risk if they have low testosterone. Speak with your doctor if any of these risk factors apply to you.

All men should follow a "healthy lifestyle" that is recommended for all women to keep bones strong especially if they are over the age of 30 when bone strength is at its peak.

How to Prevent or Treat Osteopenia

Whether or not you have diagnosed with osteopenia, all people should make sure they do the following steps to prevent any more bone loss. A diagnosis of osteopenia can be an eye-opening wake-up call to make these changes in your lifestyle.

These simple changes in lifestyle will lessen or prevent osteopenia's progression to osteoporosis. Medication is also sometimes used for a very small percentage of people who have osteopenia but we will cover the topic later on. However, medication does not mean the people should not pay attention to some simple changes in diet and lifestyle! A pill alone is not magic, it is not a cure. The following recommendations are steps incorporating lifestyle changes to prevent or treat osteopenia.

Focus on Calcium, Calcium, Calcium

Get plenty of calcium! It is the most critical mineral for bone mass. Of course, the easiest way to get it is from dairy products like milk and yogurt but you can also get it from green vegetables and calcium-enriched products. Some vegetables which are an excellent source of calcium are: kale, collard greens, broccoli, kelp, spinach and soybeans. There are many other vegetables, and fruits, that are a great source of calcium. Tofu is also a good source. And sardines (with the bones!) and salmon are a good source too. Figs have high calcium. Almonds too plus they are high in potassium. Try molasses which is high in calcium instead of honey as a sweetener.

Go darker with your greens. Bok choy, broccoli, Chinese cabbage, kale, collard greens, and turnip greens are good choices. Two lesser known nutrients that help keep bones healthy are magnesium and potassium. If you're low on magnesium, you can have problems with your vitamin D balance that helps absorb calcium. Potassium helps your body's acid that can leach out calcium in your bones that may affect your bone health. Eating a sweet potato gives you both of these nutrients.

Should you take a supplement? Talk to your doctor. If you are prescribed other medications that take away calcium, a supplement may be good for you. The best way to get calcium is from food of course. But research suggests that many of us are not getting enough calcium through diet alone. Remember too the more calcium you take at one time, the harder it is for your body to process it. Aim for 500 milligrams or less at one dosage. You may want to take a smaller amount at each meal throughout the day to add up to your total. Keep in mind, though, that you can overdo a good thing. Too much calcium may even be harmful. It's still being studied, but too much calcium could also mean a higher risk of heart disease.

So the answer as of now is if you are taking a supplement make sure you need one. You may be getting enough in your diet. It is generally believed that adults need 1,000 milligrams of calcium every day. The older you are the more you need. Women over 50 and men over 70 need 1,200 milligrams per day. But the amount may vary based on age, and other risks for osteopenia. If you think you need a supplement, always check with your doctor first.

Get Enough Vitamin D

Simply put, without enough vitamin D your body won't absorb enough calcium. If insufficient, the body will take calcium from its depository in the skeleton. This in turn, weakens existing bone and prevents any formation of strong, new bone. There are three ways to get vitamin D: though sunlight, through the diet, and through supplements.

Many people rely on the sunlight for their vitamin D. Yes, it's a great idea to get at least 5-15 minutes of sunlight every day. This is good not only for your body, which will make its own Vitamin D, but it's been proven that getting outdoors is good for your mind as well. But things like cloudy days, reduced light in winter, and the use of sun block (which is important to prevent cancer) all interfere. Add to this, dark skinned people don't make as much Vitamin D as fair skinned people do during the same time.

So, yes, it's great to get some vitamin D through the sun but it may not be enough. Diet plays a role. Eat foods like egg yolks, fatty fish like tuna, mackerel and salmon, liver, cheese, and foods fortified with Vitamin D such as dairy products, orange juice, cereals and soy milk…all high in vitamin D.

But your doctor may determine you need a supplement or are deficient. Then you need to take a supplement. A simple blood test will determine how much Vitamin D your body has. Your diet is the best way to get vitamin D. But if you still need help getting enough vitamin D (which the blood test will show), there are two kinds of supplements: D_2 (ergocalciferol), which is the type found in food, and D_3 (cholecalciferol), which is the type made from sunlight. They're produced differently, but both can raise vitamin D levels in your blood.

The recommended dietary allowance for vitamin D is 600 IU (international units) per day for adults up to age 70. People aged 71 and older should aim for 800 IU from their diet. But, like many things in life, too much vitamin D can be bad. High doses of vitamin D can raise your blood calcium level, causing damage to blood vessels, heart, and kidneys. So check with your doctor if you're getting the right amount of this essential vitamin.

Incorporate Muscle Strengthening and Weight Bearing Exercise

We all know by now that exercise is good for you. No, you don't have to join an expensive gym and as we've seen, too much can sometimes lead to osteopenia.

Develop your own exercise program. It should include both muscle strengthening and weight bearing exercise. Weight bearing means you do exercises with your feet touching the ground. This includes types that force you to work against gravity and require an upright posture. Regular exercise may prevent further bone loss and improve bone density.

Examples of muscle strengthening exercises include pushups, squats, lifting weights, or if you belong to a gym, use weight machines. Weight bearing exercises include dancing, running, walking, stair climbing, skiing and tennis. You do not have to train for a marathon! Balancing exercises are sometimes recommended too to prevent falls...and possibly breaking bones.

To go further, weight bearing exercise is any sustained activity you do against the force of gravity. High-impact or resistance workouts build more bone. Exercise that is the best for bones includes running, jumping rope, aerobic dance, basketball, tennis, baseball, skiing, skating, stair climbing, hiking, and weight lifting. Exercise that is also good but less so for bones includes walking, low-impact aerobics, most cardio machines (stair climbers, rowers, elliptical trainers, treadmill walking). The least beneficial for bones include swimming, cycling, yoga, and Pilates. But experts say if done strenuously, swimming and yoga can be better for bones. And to benefit your bones even more, divide up your exercise with short bouts of intense weight-bearing exercise. A physical therapist will work with you to decide what exercises are safe for your condition.

Loss of bone strength might start to decline earlier than you think. It slips an average rate of 1% per year after age 40. Approximately 43 million Americans are at risk for osteoporosis. If you have osteopenia, are a young adult, and are a premenopausal female, walking, jumping, or running at least 30 minutes on most days will strengthen your bones. While swimming and biking may help your heart, they don't build bones.

Regarding yoga…it can be a good exercise or bad. Contact your health care provider about engaging in yoga before beginning any practice. Only learn from an experienced, and preferably certified, teacher and be sure to explain to your teacher that you have osteopenia. If your doctor and teacher give you the go ahead, listen to your body. Do not do any weight bearing poses before you bones can handle them!

Even small increases in BMD (Bone Mineral Density) can reduce your risk for fractures later in life. As you get older, it becomes much harder for you to build bone. With age, your exercise should also emphasize muscle strengthening and balance instead. Walking is still great but now swimming and biking count too.

You can also do simple movements like toe and heel raises even while brushing your teeth. In addition to walking or other exercise, try such strengthening exercises as hip abductors (which also improve balance), prone leg lifts, squats, and forward lunges. Learn and know how to do these correctly in order not to hurt yourself. That said…don't be afraid to start slow, talk to your doctor, or get a referral to a good physical therapist. Even taking a walk around the block is a start. Just start!

Avoid Excessive Amounts of Caffeine, Salt & Alcohol

I won't tell you to avoid completely these three things that can often be a pleasure in life, caffeine, salt and alcohol. But I will tell you too much of these can mess with your bones.

Caffeine. Coffee and even chocolate (that has caffeine in it) excretes in the urine along with calcium and magnesium supplies in your body. Even though nothing has been proven, caffeine has been linked to osteopenia. Stay away too from sodas with caffeine. Many also contain phosphate acid which can decrease calcium.

If you drink alcohol, do it in moderation meaning no more than one drink per day for women and two daily drinks for men. Too much beer, wine, or liquor changes the balance of calcium in your body. Err…having too much to drink can also make you more likely to fall with a broken bone to follow!

Cut back on salt as well. Salt is known to cause excessive calcium excretion through the kidneys. Foods high in salt can thus cause the body to lose calcium and decrease bone density. And remember: it's not just table salt that increases our body's sodium. Processed food, fast food and frozen dinners are usually very high in salt.

Quit Smoking and Avoid Any Nicotine Products

We all know smoking is harmful to most if not all areas of health. This includes osteopenia. Nicotine affects how the body absorbs calcium and thus can affect bone density. Quit smoking and avoid products like chewing tobacco, nicotine gum, and patches. It can not only lead to osteopenia but osteoporosis later on.

According to the National Institute of Health, "Cigarette smoking was first identified as a risk factor for osteoporosis decades ago. Studies have shown a direct relationship between tobacco use and decreased bone density. Analyzing the impact of cigarette smoking on bone health is complicated. It is hard to determine whether a decrease in bone density is due to smoking itself or to other risk factors common among smokers. For example, in many cases smokers are thinner than nonsmokers, tend to drink more alcohol, may be less physically active, and have poor diets. Women who smoke also tend to have an earlier menopause than nonsmokers. These factors place many smokers at an increased risk for osteoporosis apart from their tobacco use.

In addition, studies on the effects of smoking suggest that smoking increases the risk of having a fracture.

As well, smoking has been shown to have a negative impact on bone healing after fracture."

Don't take the risk of getting osteopenia by smoking. If you need another excuse to quit…do it because you want to prevent osteopenia.

Adjust Prescription Medicines

This is important. Sometimes, you have another health issue and are taking medication for it that can unbeknownst to you trigger osteopenia. For example, too much thyroid medication can play a role. Other widely used medications may play a role as well. These often include steroids such as cortisone and prednisone. Anti-seizure drugs could take part. This can cause a decrease in BMD if used for a long time. They can increase fractures and eventually lead to osteoporosis.

Drugs can also include proton pump inhibitors (PPIs), some serotonin receptor inhibitors (SSRIs), thiazolidinediones (TZDs), anticonvulsants, medroxyprogesterone acetate (MPA), calcineurin inhibitors, anticoagulants and aromatese inhibitors that are used to treat breast cancer. For example, corticosteroids interferes with bone formation and stimulates bone breakdown and it has been shown 20% of all osteoporosis in the United States is due to corticosteroid use. It is a steroid replacement hormone usually used to treat cancers. Antacids reduce the production of stomach acid and weakens nutrient absorption. These have been shown to increase the risk of hip, wrist, and spine fractures. Some antidepressants are associated with a significant increase in fracture risk and often affect balance and alertness which can put you at a greater risk for falls.

While there is no need to give up these medications entirely and it is usually not recommended, you should discuss with your doctor how any of these may be affecting bone loss and adjust the dosage accordingly. Or is there an alternative? However, used over a short period these medications are not usually a problem.

Corticosteroids include:
- Beclomethasone (inhaled)
- Betamethasone (lotion or cream)
- Budesonide (capsule, inhaler, nasal spray)
- Ciclesonide (inhaled)
- Cortisone (oral, injection)
- Dexamethasone (oral)
- Ethamethasoneb (oral, injection)
- Flunisolide (inhaled)
- Fluticasone (inhaled)
- Hydrocortisone (spray, liquid, lotion, gel, cream, ointment)

- Methylpredisolone (oral)
- Mometasone (inhaled)
- Prednisone (oral)
- Triamcinolone (oral, injection)

Antacids include:
- Esomeprazole (Nexium)
- Lansoprazole (Prevacid)
- Cimetidine (Tagamet)
- Ranitidine (Zantac)

Antidepressants include:
- Citalopram (Celexa)
- Escitalopram (Lexapro)
- Fluoxetine (Prozac)
- Paroxetine (Paxil, Pexeva)
- Sertraline (Zoloft)
- Vilazodone (Viibryd)

Or another list published by Women's Health Advisor that list medications linked to bone loss includes:

- Gaviscon, Maalox, Mylanta used for heartburn or indigestion
- Phenytoin, Phenobarbital treat seizure disorder and epilepsy

- Anastrozole, Exemestane, Letrozole treat breast cancer
- Cyclosporine A, Tacrolimus used for organ transplants
- Cortisone, Prednisone to treat rheumatoid arthritis and asthma
- Esomeprazole, Omeprazole, Lansoprazole used for GERD (Gastroesophageal Reflux Disease)
- Pioglitazone, rosiglitazone used to treat Type 2 Diabetes.

This is why it's so important to list all your medications when visiting a doctor!

Many different medical specialists can treat and diagnose osteopenia. These include a primary care provider, rheumatologist, endocrinologist, and gynecologist. Others can as well because they are dispensing medication that may predispose you to osteopenia. And osteoporosis. So speak to your practitioner about perhaps taking a less bone-damaging alternative.

Follow an Osteopenia Diet and Maintain a Healthy Weight

Overall, you should consume a diet rich in vegetables, fruit, sea vegetables and other plant foods. Aim towards an alkaline diet versus an acidic diet. Cruciferous vegetables are supposed to be among the best options for promoting alkalinity. Processed oils, nuts, refined grains, alcohol, and animal protein are believed to have a net acidic effect.

It's good for your health in general and will lower your sodium if you eat unprocessed and whole foods. It's best to avoid or limit any deli meats, fast foods, fried foods, canned foods, salty condiments or sauces and frozen meals. Limit sugary products too. This includes sweetened drinks.

Sometimes, especially women, limit their calories to achieve a low body fat percentage or desired weight. But undereating if done for many years can result in osteopenia with a host of problems. Therefore, it's important to eat an adequate number of calories to fuel your body's processes. However, maintain a healthy weight! The other end of the scale…obesity can increase inflammation and contribute to hormonal changes that can damage bones. And if you're not obese, it's just easier to be active and exercise.

You must make sure you are getting adequate nutrients to fuel your body. This of course includes calcium and vitamin D. But other nutrients in order to prevent bone disorders include iron, vitamin C, and magnesium. Iron deficiency or anemia, is often a risk factor for osteopenia because iron is essential for vitamin D metabolism. Vitamin C plays a role in collagen formation. Collagen is a protein that provides structure to much of your body, including bones, skin, tendons and ligaments. Vitamin C also helps in stimulating cells that build bones, boosts calcium absorption, and aids in vitamin D working.

Magnesium rich foods include leafy greens like spinach, pumpkin seeds, yogurt, black beans, and almonds. Vitamin C foods include: citrus fruits, berries, peppers, kiwi, broccoli and kale. Food that provide iron include beef, lamb, chicken, turkey, fish, eggs, and nuts. Collagen can be found naturally in bone broth (which is high in calcium too!) or can be taken in powder form or as a supplement. Most people can prevent vitamin B12 deficiency by eating enough meat, poultry, seafood, dairy products, and eggs. But consider taking Vitamin B12 supplements. Supplements are especially good for the elderly or vegetarians. According to research studies, vitamin B12 is a benefit for nerve health but it may also be a benefit for bone health.

Always discuss taking any supplement with your doctor first!

Medication for Osteopenia

In a very few cases, your doctor may prescribe a medication to lower your chances of getting osteoporosis. Or, if you've already broken a bone, your practitioner may believe lifestyle changes along with medicine is needed. Drugs for bone disorders aren't usually a cure as the condition tends to worsen with age. However, medication may substantially slow down bone loss.

If this is the case, your doctor will prescribe three categories of medication. However, you may want to discuss with your medical practitioner, why you need the medication and cannot slow down bone loss naturally without medication.

The three categories are:

1. Bisphosphonate medications which include alendronate (Fosamax), ibandronate (Boniva),

risedronic (Actonel), and zoledronic (Reclast) acid. Most are pills but Reclast is an injection.

2. Anabolic medications usually called teriparatide (Forteo). According to WebMD, "it is the only osteoporosis medicine approved by the FDA that rebuilds bone…is self-injected into the skin. Because long-term safety is not yet established, it is only FDA-approved for 24 months of use.

3. Raloxifene (Evista) can prevent and treat osteoporosis. According to the National Osteoporosis Foundation it "is approved for the prevention and treatment of osteoporosis in postmenopausal women. It is in a class of drugs called estrogen agonists/antagonists that have been developed to provide the beneficial effects of estrogens without all of the potential disadvantages. It is neither an estrogen nor a hormone. Raloxifene is sometimes called a selective estrogen receptor modulator (SERM)."

As with any drug, all these have their own risks and possible side effects. So make sure to talk to your doctor about these before you take any of them. (Remember my mom couldn't take Fosamax!). For example, a Forteo injection causes abnormally rapid growth of bone cells, resulting in a very frightening side effect: osteosarcoma, a form of bone cancer. The relatively new Forteo was approved by the FDA.

"FDA approval" just means that the FDA has decided the benefits of the approved item outweigh the potential risks for the item's planned use. And there are many questions about the FDA being tied to "Big Pharma" even contributing to generic drugs being distributed. To have more unhealthy people means more drug sales to "Big Pharma". It's a business after all. There are websites that say never take osteoporosis drugs even if you have been diagnosed with osteoporosis let alone osteopenia!

So, it comes down to you as an individual unfortunately. We are all different. Drugs will affect us differently. Do you trust your doctor's advice too?

Physicians should explain all the side effects and risks to you if you take a drug. Yet, every story has two sides. If the side effects are very rare, you may want to consider taking medication for the good of your bones. Whatever you decide, it pays to be an educated patient or patient advocate.

A Note on Dental X-Rays

Many people see their dentist much more often than their doctor. Dental X-rays can often be used as a screening tool for osteoporosis from those with normal bone density. Dentists are in a very good position to tell patients to discuss osteopenia with a doctor or whether to get a DXA scan. Dental concerns that may indicate low bone density include loose teeth, gums detaching from the teeth or receding guns, and ill-fitting or loose dentures. So if your dentist encourages you to talk to your doctor about bone loss, make an appointment and do it!

Can Osteopenia Be Reversed?

You definitely should know the root cause of your osteopenia. Everybody's bones get weaker as they get older. But certain choices and habits speed up the process as we've seen.

A research study found that how fast osteopenia progresses depends on how severe the osteopenia was when it was discovered. So, the worse the osteopenia, the shorter the development time to osteoporosis.

In other words, sometimes but very infrequently, osteopenia will normalize on follow-up testing. This is more common in certain situations, such as when only mild osteopenia is found on the initial bone density test. For example, when mild osteopenia is caused by significant vitamin D deficiency, and the vitamin D deficiency is treated, then the osteopenia may reverse. However, remember osteopenia can be reversed in only a minority of people! More often, osteopenia does not reverse. But it can always be lessened.

In general, low BMD progresses over time. It is a fact that as you age your bones get weaker. It's best to know how to treat osteopenia to avoid ever, ever getting osteoporosis. Concentrate on treating osteopenia…don't worry about it turning into osteoporosis…and it may just get better and never worse!

May is National Osteoporosis Month

Hopefully, you will never get osteoporosis even after having been diagnosed with osteopenia. But I wanted you to know of this month in case you may want to volunteer in your community to help make others aware of the disease.

For The American Academy of Orthopedic Surgeons fairly recently conducted a study saying "that even though osteoporosis can lead to debilitating fractures, pain, spinal problems, loss of independence, and even death, many at-risk seniors have little knowledge about the disease." "Many people who sustain a fracture don't connect it to osteoporosis," said study author Dr. Angela M. Cheung of the University Health Network/Mount Sinai Hospital Osteoporosis Program in Toronto, Ontario. Cheung points out in contrast, "A person who has a heart attack knows that there's a problem with his or her heart, but a person who fractures thinks, 'The floor was slippery' or 'I'm clumsy' and doesn't look at it as a symptom of a more serious medical condition."

Now that you're somewhat educated yourself, it may be time to educate others on osteopenia and how it can relate to osteoporosis.

Final Words

Remember: osteopenia is not a disease but it can be a precursor to osteoporosis. But with healthy lifestyle changes (and rarely medication) you can prevent it from it ever going that far. It's never too early to make these changes...even for a teen-aged girl who hasn't been diagnosed. So start today...you can totally prevent or successfully treat osteopenia!

Made in the USA
Coppell, TX
01 February 2024

28477717R00036